Move!
You Are Not A Tree

The Journey to a Back Pain-Free Life and Optimal Health

Patrice St. Claire
MP Publishing

Table of Contents

Introduction

The human body is designed to move as it is the essence of being alive. For thousands of years, that's exactly what humans did. Our strong legs and subtly curved spines are not created for us to be passive; instead, these are intricately designed to help us stand upright and move about our lives. However, in the mid-20th century, rapid technological advances—TVs, computers, smartphones, the Internet, etc.—began chipping away at physical activity, and as technology did more of the heavy lifting and jobs that require physical labor, people became increasingly sedentary.

Look around you. Chances are you're in an environment that requires sitting for a long period of time. The majority of our workplaces, homes, schools, and public spaces decrease activity and movement, and the low-intensity or non-exercise activities—standing and walking—that are so vital to health has been replaced with sedentary ones—binge-watching, video game playing, driving automobiles, web surfing, and reading.

The awareness of the harmful impacts of inactivity is increasing, yet we disregard this fact and take our systems for granted. That's why progress has been surprisingly slow and difficult. The unfortunate reality is that many daily activities and social norms involve the use of chairs.

It's high time to activate our offices, schools, and homes. When reading this book, therefore, make sure to take a break every 30 minutes, stretch or just walk around for 3-5 minutes then go back to reading.

WHAT YOU NEED TO KNOW

The Health Hazards of Prolonged Sitting

Every time we think we have a handle on all the things that are harmful for us, another one is added to the list. A couple of years ago, researchers put inactivity on the list of major health risks. A professor of medicine at Harvard Medical School, Dr. I-Min Lee says, "Everybody knows smoking is bad for your health. But what is not common knowledge is that physical inactivity is as powerful a risk factor as smoking." Dr. Lee was one of the first to identify inactivity as a health hazard as she has studied the outcomes of exercise for more than a decade.

By this time, you already know that sitting too much is bad, not only for your back but also for your whole body. But what exactly happens when you sit for long hours every day? Let's dig deep on how your body is affected.

Bad Back

- **Inflexible Spine:** Being active results in soft discs between vertebrae to expand and contract like sponges, soaking up fresh blood and nutrients. But prolonged sitting causes discs to be squeezed unevenly. Collagen hardens around ligaments and tendons.

- **Disk Damage:** People who sit for long hours are at greater risk for herniated lumbar disks. A muscle called the psoas travels through the abdominal cavity and, when it constricts, pulls the upper lumbar spine forward. Rather than the upper-body weight being distributed along the arch of the spine, it rests entirely on the ischial tuberosity (sitting bones).

Organ Damage

- **Heart Disease:** During a long sit, muscle burn less fat and blood flows more sluggishly, which allow fatty acids to more easily clog the heart. Sitting for long periods of time has been associated to high blood pressure and increased cholesterol, and people with the most sedentary time are more susceptible to have cardiovascular disease than those with the least.

- **Over Productive Pancreas:** The pancreas produces insulin, a hormone that carries glucose to cells for energy, and keeps our blood sugar from getting too high (hyperglycemia) or too low (hypoglycemia). However, cells in idle muscles don't respond as readily to insulin, so the pancreas produces more and more, which can give birth to diabetes and other diseases. In 2011, research found a decline in insulin response after an all-day sitting.

- **Colon Cancer:** Researches have found that chronic sitters have a greater risk for colon, breast, and endometrial cancers. The root is unclear, but one theory is that excess insulin stimulates cell growth. Another is that regular movement promotes natural antioxidants that kill cell-damaging— and potentially cancer-causing — free radicals.

Trouble at the Top

- **Foggy Brain:** Moving muscles pump fresh blood and oxygen into the brain and trigger the release of all kinds of brain- and mood-enhancing chemicals. When we are passive for a long time, everything slows, including brain function.

- **Strained Neck:** If most of your sitting occurs at a desk at work, craning your neck forward toward a keyboard or tilting your head to cradle a phone while typing can damage the cervical vertebrae and result in permanent imbalances.

- **Sore Shoulders and Back:** The neck doesn't slouch alone. Slumping forward overextends both your shoulder and back muscles, especially the trapezius that joins the neck and shoulders.

Muscle Degeneration

- **Mushy Abs:** When you stand, move, or even sit up straight, abdominal muscles keep you upright.

When you slump in a chair, however, they go unused. Tight back muscles and weak abs form a posture-wrecking alliance, which can lead to exaggeration of the spine's natural arch, a condition called hyperlordosis, or swayback.

- **Tight Hips:** Flexible hips help keep you balanced, but chronic sitters so rarely stretch the hip flexor muscles in front that they become short and tight, restricting range of motion and stride length. Researchers have found that reduced hip mobility is a main cause elderly people tend to fall.

- **Limp Glutes:** Sitting requires your glutes to do absolutely nothing, and they get accustomed to it. Soft glutes hurt your stability, your ability to push off and to keep a powerful stride.

Leg Disorders

- **Poor Circulation in Legs:** Prolonged sitting slows blood circulation, which causes fluid to pool in the legs. Problems range from varicose veins and swollen ankles to dangerous blood clots called deep vein thrombosis (DVT).

- **Soft Bones:** Weight-lifting activities including walking and running help hip and lower-body bones to grow thicker, denser, and stronger. Scientists partially attribute the recent surge in cases of osteoporosis to sedentary lifestyle.

Back Pain Risk Factors

Whether you're an elite athlete, or a weekend warrior, or somewhere in between, chances are back ache will hit you sooner or later, as well. Here's why: Everyday activities that you do without thinking — slipping on a pair of shoes, sitting at the computer, crawling into bed at night — can make or break the health of your spine.

Most aches are caused by sprains (damage to the tough fibrous tissue, or ligaments, which is located at where your vertebrae connect to joints) or strains (injured muscles or tendons). These injuries are typically brought on by overuse, excessive lifting, a new activity, or an accident. Other times, a compressed or pinched nerve, including a herniated disk, is to blame for the pain.

If you belong to the 80 percent of the population that regularly suffers from back ache, take heart: One-third of aches due to a sprain or a strain relieve in a week without medical intervention (the remainder may take up to eight weeks). But unless you do some spine tuning — strengthening your back through exercise and developing healthier habits — your chance of a recurrence within six months are about one in three. You can have a back-pain free life by avoiding these seven spinal sins:

You're a screen queen.

Are you a screen queen, spending all day hunched over to your computer or just obsessed with your smart phone? Either way, you are putting so much stress in your spine, thus having a greater risk to suffer back problems. Nine hours — that's how long the average person consumes slouched huddled over in front of a screen each day.

You ignore your core.

When you hear the word core, having six-pack abs comes into mind. But your core is composed of much more: Back, pelvic, side, and buttock muscles all work together, along with your abs, which enable you to twist, bend, rotate, and stand upright.

You sleep on your stomach.

Sleep allows your body to heal and recharge for the day ahead. However, your sleeping position could be one of the causes of lower back pain, particularly sleeping on your stomach. Women who practice the art of stomach sleeping may snore less, but it could be problematic on the back. This is because bedtime belly flop puts stress on joints and muscles, while sleeping on your side or back keeps your spine neutral and elongated.

You like to light up.

Cigarettes aren't just hell on your heart and lungs. Smokers have a higher probability of recurring back problems; as nicotine limits blood flow to vertebrae and disks, hence they may age and break down more quickly. Moreover, it also interferes with the body's ability to absorb and use calcium, producing osteoporosis-related bone and back problems.

You're an emotional mess.

It's no secret that struggling with pain can take a toll on your mental well-being, and researches have shown that people who suffer from back pain are more likely to have depression. In addition, doctors are now discovering that the reverse may be true as well: In study conducted from the University of Alberta in Canada, people with major depression were four times as likely to develop disabling low-back and neck pain. Some scientists postulated that poor coping skills associated with depression, including withdrawing or avoiding problems, may trigger the release of the stress hormone cortisol, resulting in back and shoulder muscles to tense up and spasm.

You're a slave to fashion.

Sure, sky-high stilettos are a no-no, but it turns out that flats can be of trouble, too, as they offer little to no arch support. Wearing them regularly can lead to back problems and back pains that hamper your daily routine. Alternate styles throughout the week — from high to low, sandals to sneakers — and avoid wearing a particular pair every day. Your purse could also be a culprit of back, neck, and shoulder pain, especially if it's huge and you're lugging it on one shoulder. Try using a tote with a wide, padded strap; carry it messenger style; and reduce the load. According to the American Chiropractic Association, the maximum weight of bag should be less than 10 percent of your body weight.

degree of pain experienced such as mood, stress levels, fitness, fear of injury, and individual coping mechanisms.

Myth: Being overweight doesn't contribute to back pain.

Fact: Extra body weight compresses the spine and squeezes intervertebral disks, making an overweight individual more susceptible to painful back conditions. Moreover, high amounts of belly fat can result in poor posture and slouching causing back pain, as extra pounds put stress on your back. Majority of the people who are out of shape suffered back pain, mainly weekend warriors who push themselves hard after sitting around all week.

Myth: Exercise is bad for back pain.

Fact: This is a big one. Many people who are in pain are afraid of exercise and avoid it as they think it may lead to more problems. Actually, regular exercise helps to keep you and your body fit and healthy, keeping you from having back pain or reducing discomfort. It relaxes muscle tension, promotes good mood, and strengthens the immune system. Even doctors may recommend exercise for people who have recently hurt their lower back. They usually start with gentle movements and gradually build up the intensity. Once the immediate pain goes away, an exercise plan can help keep it from coming back.

The Red Flags

While some back pains resolve naturally in a couple of weeks, other needs immediate medical attention. Doctors look for certain factors called Red Flags that could determine that something is going on in the back that could cause concern. Moreover, other considerations called Yellow Flags can be signs of increased risk of back pain becoming chronic.

Anyone with these symptoms with back pain should seek immediate medical help, as they could point to the development of a rare condition, that affects the bundle of nerve roots (cauda equina) at the lower (lumbar) end of the spinal cord, called **cauda equina syndrome**:

- Difficulty passing urine
- Having a bowel movement
- Numbness in the "saddle area"
- Progressive weakness in the legs
- Severe and continuous abdominal and low back pain

There are several warning signs, known as red flag signs, that may signify that your back pain is caused by a more serious condition that needs immediate medical care. These include:

- A fever of 100.4°F (38°C) or above
- Unexplained weight loss
- Constant back pain that does not go away after lying down
- Swelling of the back
- Numbness around your genitals, buttocks, or back passage
- Pain caused by a recent trauma or injury to your back
- Pain in your chest or high up in your back
- Pain down your legs and below the knees
- Inability to pass urine
- Loss of bowel control
- Loss of bladder control
- Pain that is worse at night

Red Flags

- Previous history malignancy (however long ago)

- Age of onset is less than 16 or more than 55 years old
- Recent history of violent trauma
- Constant and progressive non mechanical pain (no relief with bed rest)
- Structural deformity
- Unexplained weight loss
- Thoracic pain
- Prolonged use of corticosteroids
- Drug abuse, immunosuppression, HIV
- Systemically unwell
- Widespread neurological symptoms (including cauda equine syndrome)
- Fever

WHAT YOU NEED TO DO

Keep Fit at Your Workplace

Cases of work-related disorders are not isolated to heavy manufacturing or construction. They arise in all kinds of industries and work environments, even office spaces which is defined by the use of chairs. Study shows that poor posture, repetitive motion, and staying in the same position can lead to or worsen musculoskeletal disorders. These are normal in a desk job. An analysis of job industry trends over the past 50 years showed that at least 8 in 10 American workers are desk potatoes. The good news is that moving or stretching is a buildable habit.

So what's a worker chained to his or her desk to do? Fortunately, strength exercises, short bouts of aerobics, and stretching in between conference calls and group chats can improve fitness levels and overall health. While these deskercises, or desk exercises for the cubicle-bound, won't promise six-pack abs or Olympic mile times, they can prevent and reverse your back pain. But no one wants to do a mile run or anything else that will get their work clothes sweaty, hence these simple exercises can keep your clothes neat and still get your heart rate up.

Stretch at Your Desk

The Letter "O"

Start with your left hand, spread out and straighten your fingers. Then, curve all of your fingers inward until they meet. Your fingers should form the shape of an "O." Hold this position for a few seconds. Then relax and straighten your fingers again. Repeat this stretch a few times a day on each hand. Do this stretch whenever your hands feel stiff or achy.

Shrug

Raise both your shoulders, reaching your ears until there's a slight tension build in your neck and shoulders. Hold this feeling of tension for about 3-5 seconds, then release and relax your shoulders into their normal position. Repeat this for about 2-3 times. Good to use at the first signs of tension or tightness or in the shoulder and neck area.

Twist and Turn

You have a bad posture.

As we discussed earlier, slouching not only makes us look unattractive but also causes back, knee, shoulder and hips relate problems. Poor body posture strains our muscles and elevates stress on our spine. In the long run, bad posture can also interfere with the anatomical characteristics of spine. Poor sleeping posture, spending too much time commuting, or sitting for too long can affect our stance and intensify back pains.

Back pain is one of the most common, and worst, pains we have to cope with as we get older. But it doesn't only affect the mature, it can happen at any age, any place and any time, for various reasons. It is also second to the common cold for being the reason employees miss work.

As a common problem, many people will suggest many solutions or you will find health information which is available online, so it's good to know in advance which are legitimate or bogus. Hence, it's important to weed through the clutter and identify the facts from the common misconceptions about back problems. Here is the list that will make that clearer:

Myth: Strong painkillers are the answer.

Fact: Many people think strong pain requires a strong painkiller. That is wrong. If you have a new episode of back pain, you should start with a simple painkiller. Strong pain killers including those containing an opioid do give a little more pain relief, but not a lot more, and they have greater potential for side effects. Continuous or persistent back pain is different. Long term use of strong painkillers is scarcely a good management option, especially if that is the only treatment. There are now some newer pain management programs that can relieve people with persistent back pain come off strong painkillers without making their pain worse.

Myth: Scans and x-rays are needed.

Fact: In the majority of cases of low back pain, scans and x-rays are unnecessary. Every year large sums of money are wasted on inessential X-rays and scans for low back pain. In only a small number of cases will these tests actually show something truly important, which contribute to better management of the problem. Even adults with no previous record of low back pain will reveal normal "wear and tear" on these scans. A simple clinical test will determine the minority of people for whom scans are required.

Myth: Sitting upright prevents back pain.

Fact: While sitting hunched over does cause damage to your back, sitting upright for long periods can also be a strain on your back. In order to reduce the damage caused by prolonged sitting, you should lean back once in a while with your feet on the floor and allow your back curve slightly. Moreover, try standing for part of the day, perhaps while you're on the phone or reading.

Myth: No heavy lifting.

Fact: In most cases concerned with back pain, it's not how much you lift, it's how you do it. A correct lift is as follows: squat close to it with your back straight and head up, stand and use your legs to push up the load while your arms to hold it close to your middle. Your back won't hurt as long as you don't involve it in picking up anything that might be too heavy for you, which you shouldn't.

Myth: Bed rest is the best treatment.

Fact: Bed rest, once a key part of treating sore backs, has a limited role in healing back pains. In very small doses, bed rest can give you a break when standing or sitting results in severe pain. However, staying in the same position for a long time can make the pain worse and the pressure on the back and spine increase.

Myth: Back pain is only caused by injury.

Fact: Disc degeneration, diseases, infections, inherited conditions, and even sedentary lifestyle can make your back hurt, too.

Myth: Surgery is a must.

Fact: Only a tiny proportion of people with back pain need surgery. Majority of those who have back pain can deal with it by staying active, having a growing understanding of what pain means, and determining the factors which contribute to their pain. This should aid them continue their usual daily tasks, without having to resort to surgery. On average, the outcomes for spinal surgery are no better in the medium and long-term than non-surgical interventions, such as exercise.

Myth: The more back pain, the more spine is damaged.

Fact: More pain does not always mean more damage. People who have similar back injuries can experience different levels of pain. Many factors can contribute to the

This is a good stretch for the side hip, lower and middle back. Sit with your right leg bent over left leg, then rest your left elbow or forearm on the outside of the upper thigh of the right leg. Then, apply some controlled and steady pressure toward the left with the elbow or forearm. As you do this, look over your right shoulder to get the stretch feeling. Do both sides. Hold for 15 seconds.

Say Aah

This stretch may cause people around you to think you are very queer indeed, but it is helpful as you often find a lot of tension in your face due to eye strain. Raise your eyebrows and open your eyes as wide as possible. At the same time, open your mouth to stretch the muscles around your nose and chin, then stick your tongue out. Hold this stretch for about 5-10 seconds. Caution: If you have clicking or popping noises when you open your mouth, you should ask your dentist first before doing this stretch.

Look Around

Begin with head in a comfortable, upright position. Slowly tilt your head to the right side, stretching the muscles on side of your neck. Hold position for about 10-20 seconds. Feel a good and even stretch, but do not overstretch. Then tilt head to left side and stretch. Repeat for about 2-3 times in each side.

Rubber Neck

Sit up tall and straight, tilt your left ear towards your left shoulder (you don't have to touch it!). Hold stretch for 8 seconds. Do the same thing with your right ear to your right shoulder. Repeat for 5 times.

Chest Opener

Interlace your fingers behind your head, keeping your elbows straight out at sides with your upper body in upright position. Then, pull your shoulder blades toward each other until you feel a tension in your upper back and shoulder blades. Hold this feeling of mild tension for about 7-10 seconds, then release. Repeat for several times. Do this when upper back and shoulders are tight or tense.

Bobble Head

With a stable and upright sitting position, slowly place your chin toward your left shoulder, creating a tension on the right side of your neck. Hold position for 10-20 seconds. Repeat twice for each side.

Crane

Gently tilt your head forward to stretch the back of the neck. Hold the stretch for about 5-10 seconds. Repeat 3-5 times. Hold the stretch where the tension feels good and not to the point of pain.

Reach and Bend

Extend your left arm over your head, and then reach out as far as you can to the right, gently bending over. Hold stretch for a few seconds and do it the other way.

Reach for the Stars

Clasp your hands firmly as you interlace your fingers together then reach up towards the sky, as high as you can but still relaxing, stretching your arms out with your palms towards the ceiling. Hold for about 10-20 seconds. Repeat 3 times.

Toe-Toucher

Sit upright and stretch your left arm as high as you can towards the ceiling. Straighten your right leg out and raise it up as you bring your left arm down and try to touch your left foot. Repeat for about 8–10 times on each side.

Knee Hugger

With a bent knee, lift your left leg up and grab it with your arms, pulling it in as close to your chest as you can. Hold position for about 5–10 seconds and make sure and do it on the right side, as well.

Backward Clap

Put your hands behind your back and interlace your fingers. Slowly turn your elbows inward while you straighten your arms. Hold position for about 5-15 seconds. Do twice. This is an excellent stretch for shoulders and arms. This is best done when you find yourself slumping forward from your shoulders and can be done at any time.

Wall-Assisted Calf Stretch

Stand a little less than arm's distance from wall for solid support and lean on it. Keeping feet parallel, step left foot forward until toes touch wall in front of you. Bend your left knee and lean forward to place hands on wall, keeping back leg straight and pressing heel into the ground. Hold position for 30 seconds and switch legs.

Exercise at Your Desk

Walk/Jog/Run in Place

This is easy, as all you need is enough open space so that you don't bump into your coworkers. Also, you are in control of the intensity based on the pace you choose. Want an even bigger challenge? Bring your knees up to waist level. Do this for 30–45 seconds. Repeat 3–5 times.

Push-Ups

Hold your horses! Don't do it in your office floor! There are options besides the floor. The alternatives are to do them on the wall or on the edge of your desk. However, if you are going to do them against the wall, make sure it's not a cubicle wall; otherwise you could end up on your colleague's desk. Do 10 reps. Repeat 3 times.

Squats

From your chair, stand up, and sit back down. Repeat 10 more times. Simple!

Tricep Dips

Tricep dips can be done pretty much anywhere. Position your butt on the edge of a stable desk, then put your palms on the edge of the desk on either side of you. Keep your feet together and bend your arms to about a 90-degree angle, straighten, and repeat! Do this 20 times. You can also use your chair if it doesn't have wheels on it.

Star Jumps

Stand with your feet together, hands at your sides,. Jump and extend your legs to shoulder-width apart, whilst bringing your arms together over your head. Do this for 5-10 minutes; you can have breaks in between.

Calf Raises

Starting with your feet together, stand behind your chair and hold on for support, and rise up on your tippy toes. Hold position for about 10 seconds, and then release and repeat. It's a simple exercise that will leave you feeling stretched and revived.

Glute Squeezes

Sit in your chair with your feet extended in front of you. Simply squeeze your glutes as hard as you can. Clench for 2 seconds, release then repeat the squeeze. Complete these 20 short clenches and then squeeze and hold position for 30 seconds. Repeat the sequence several times throughout the day.

Shoulder Press

Look around the office and search for an old phone book, a ream of paper, or your tumbler full of water, something that weighs a few pounds. Hold it at shoulder height and then raise it all the way overhead. Do it for 10 reps. Repeat 3 times.

Wall Sit

Stand with your back against the wall, bend your knees, and slowly lower yourself, sliding down the wall until your thighs are parallel to the floor. Hold position for 60 seconds. If you want an even bigger challenge, cross your right ankle over your left knee for a one-legged wall sit. Hold for 15 seconds, then switch.

Lunge

You can either do this exercise at your desk, or you could lunge down the hall to the coffee or printer and back. Position one leg forward with knee bent and food flat on the ground, whilst the other leg is positioned behind; as if you were going to propose to a co-worker. Do 10 times on each leg.

Leave Your Desk

Park Farther Away

Parking so close to the office or gym means that you are missing a great opportunity to add more steps to your day. While parking farther and walking to the entrance of your office is an easy way to incorporate more physical activity in your daily routine.

Take the Stairs

Do you hate making small talk while you're on the elevator? Take the stairs instead. Using the stairs are a fantastic way to increase your heart rate and tone up those legs.

Do It Yourself

Having an assistant may be an advantage of your job, but if you'll get your own coffee and walk over to the printer more often, you will be spending less time sitting.

Stand Up

If you have to be on the phone a lot, what better time to stand up, go for a walk, or do some stretches. Seriously, go ahead, the person on the other end of the line can't see you!

Take a Walk Break

Spend your break wisely by taking a walk. Use a fitness tracker to see how many steps you can get. If it's nice outside, go get some fresh air especially when you're surrounded by trees. You may also find someone to go with you to share this daily routine and book with.

Live Chat

In lieu of picking up the phone or sending an email over to Drew in IT department, you actually go and pay him a visit? You get to move more, and I'm sure Drew will appreciate the company once in a while.

Walk and Talk

Why not have a walking meeting next time rather than sitting in a cold conference room at a table with cold coffee and stale donuts? And because exercise improves brain function—particularly creativity—, you may come up with some of your best ideas!

Commute Differently

If you reside in a city and use public transportation, try getting off the train or the bus a stop or two before your usual destination and hence getting some extra steps in. If you live close enough to work, forget the bus, hop on your bike or put on your sneakers, and hit the pavement.

Drink More Water

Hit two birds with one stone by filling up your tumbler more often at the office. Add even more steps to your daily routine with the extra bathroom trips. If you're bladder is far from exploding, use a restroom on a different floor and take the stairs to reach it.

Mr./Ms. Congeniality

Offer to make coffee for your nearby co-worker. You'll be adding more steps to your daily routine as you'll have to walk to the coffee room and then to their desks.

You now have an arsenal of tips and tricks you can apply to help optimize your health, and reverse or prevent the consequences of sedentary lifestyle. Ideally you should get up from your desk at least once an hour, even if it's not exercises to do at your desk. Schedule or set an alarm to remind you to stop squinting at that Excel worksheet and get up and move. Work can provide plenty of opportunities for walking. You just need to seek them out, and of course, apply them!

Instead of staying camped out on your couch while watching TV, make us of commercial breaks as more time for physical activity. Standing up and doing something during commercial breaks or even while your favorite show is on—whether it be folding clothes, doing a few sit-ups or push-ups, or any number of other activities—will limit or break up the extra sedentary time that leads to accrue during most, if not all, screen-based activities. The following activities provide simple and perfect ways to help you convert your sedentary lifestyle at home, without much effort.

Stretches

Hip Opener

Sit on the edge of a bench, table, or bed. Lie down on your back, your entire lower back should be in contact with the surface. Bring your right knee to your chest both hands and extend left leg so it hangs freely. Hold stretch for at least 20-30 seconds, then relax and lower your right knee to the starting position. Repeat with the left leg. Repeat 2-4 times with each leg.

Side Stretch

Lie on the floor on your left side with your forearm supporting you. Bend your right leg and move it up toward your stomach as far as you can without moving your left leg. Plant your right foot on the floor. Slowly raise your upper body so that your left arm is straight. Stop when you feel a mild tension in the left side of your waist. Hold stretch for about 20-30 seconds. Do 2 sets on each side.

L-Stand

Stand facing a table or surface that's about as high as the top of your thighs. Lift your left knee and raise your ankle so the entire outside of your leg is resting on the table. Your left leg should form an L shape and be in line with your hip. Bend your lower back and tilt your upper body forward. Hold position for about 20-30 seconds. Do 2 sets on each side.

Frog Press

Begin with lying face down with your head on hands, your legs should be wider than hip-distance, your knees bent 90 degrees and the soles of your feet together. Lift your thighs off floor, hold for 5-7 seconds, then relax to floor. Repeat 12 times.

Foldover Stretch

Stand upright with feet hip-width apart, knees slightly bent, arms by sides. Exhale as you tilt forward from hips, lowering your head toward floor, while keeping your head, neck and shoulders relaxed. Wrap arms around backs of legs and hold anywhere from 1-2 minutes. Bend knees and roll up slowly to release.

Butterfly Stretch

Start with sitting on the floor with the soles of your feet together and knees bent out to sides. Hold your feet with your hands. Slowly lower your body toward your feet, going only as far as you can. Hold position for 1-2 minutes. Slowly release. If you find this stretch uncomfortable, elevate your hips onto a couple of blankets or a pillow, and then retry.

Standing Thigh Release

Stand upright with your feet together and arms by sides. Bring your left heel toward butt and grasp the top of your left foot using your left hand. Extend right arm overhead (or place on chair) to keep your balance. Grasp your left foot with your hand to increase stretch along front of thigh. Hold position for a minute, release, then switch sides and repeat.

Exercises

Kick Back

Stand on your right leg. As you inhale, bring your left knee to your chest while crunching your torso forward. As you exhale, jump, and kick your leg back to extend your torso, bringing your arms back, too. Do 2 sets of 40 seconds on each leg.

Fire Hydrant

Begin standing with your feet together and your knees slightly bent. Lean forward and put your hands above your knees, pulling your abs inward. Raise and bend your left leg, bringing it behind you and then toward you in large circular motions. Do 15 reps on each leg.

Inchworm to Grasshopper

Get into a push-up position. With stable arms and shoulders, jump and bring each shin to the opposite arm. Do 2 sets of 10 reps.

Tap It Out

Begin in a yoga chair position, squat your butt to the back and bring your arms straight above your head. As you bring one leg out to the side, bring your arms down, keeping them bent at your shoulders. Bring your leg back in then return to the yoga chair position. Repeat on the other side. Do this for 40 seconds for 4 reps.

Flying Passé

Do a side plank position, using one arm to hold yourself up and your other arm bent at your hip. Bend the leg that's closest to the ground and bring it straight out behind you, twisting your hips. Bring your leg back in. Do 3 sets of 10 on each side.

Indoor and Outdoor Activities

Make your grocery trip a healthy one.

When you go to the grocery store, get the most mileage out of your errand by walking up and down each aisle, nook, and corner. However, avoid sections that could tempt you to pick up junk food, as it can completely obliterate any benefits of walking a few extra steps! Skip this if you have a spending problem.

Play with your kids.

Nowadays, kids are also prone to having a sedentary lifestyle as they seem to play more video games than outdoor games like we did when we were younger. So take your kids out to the park and throw the ball around, play tag or hide and seek, etc. Doing so is good for all of you.

Put on your favorite music and dance.

This is a fun way to burn calories and unwind at the end of a busy day. And a good trip down the memory lane for those of us who have not done it in a pretty long time!

Choose active entertainment over passive ones.

Rather than going for a movie, playing regular video games, or meeting friends for a cup of coffee, choose to go play tennis with some friends, play with a Wii, or catch up over a sunset walk.

Choose active vacations.

Vacations are also great opportunities to be even further active. Rather than planning a retreat to a spa, plan to revitalize your mind and body by hiking. Instead of taking in a new city by driving around, walk the downtown area. When golfing, skip the golf cart and walk the course. If staying at a resort, take advantage of their pool and exercise facility.

III. BONUS TIPS TO EASE YOUR BACK PAIN

Customize Your Desk and Chair

Dr. Scott Donkin, founder of Occupational Health and Wellness Solutions consults workplaces on safety, health, and ergonomic issue. He then postulates that the act of leaning forward in your chair crushes the disks in your lower back and puts strain on your neck and shoulders. San Francisco State University's Dr. Erik Peper recommends the following tips to help yourself naturally lean back as you work.

- Support the natural structure and curve of your spine! Office chairs must have lumbar support, a natural forward curve at belly button level. To achieve this effect, you can also put a pillow or rolled up towel behind your back.

- Adjust the height of your chair so you can keep your feet flat on the floor and your knees arch at 90-degree angles. For extra support, you can also rest your feet on a footrest. Crossing your legs tightly minimizes circulation in your legs and leads to varicose veins, which look dark blue on your skin!

- Remove or lower the height of the armrests so your arms are at 90-degree angles. This will keep you to hold your shoulders low, which your upper back will thank you for.

- Keep your monitor about an arm's length away with the top of the monitor at about or slightly below eye level. Instead of leaning forward, the latter advice will encourage you to sit back and reduces neck strain. Adjust the lighting to lessen strain on the eyes if you find yourself squinting at your monitor.

Optimize Your Phone Calls

As we discussed earlier, many people tuck their phone between their head and shoulder to free up their hands while talking, which results to strained neck and shoulders. Try these alternatives to avoid tucking your phone during your conversations.

- Use an earphones or a speakerphone if your conversation takes more than 5 minutes or you need to take notes during the call.
- Hold the phone in your hand and switch between your right and left sides throughout the conversation.

Ice it

Applying an ice pack to the painful area as it can help keep inflammation at bay and relieve discomfort, as it lessens the ability of nerves to send pain signals to the brain. Ice it by putting ice cubes in a plastic bag, then apply the bag on top of a thin towel that has been placed on the skin to avoid ice burn. Leave the ice pack on for no more than 20 minutes, take it off for 30 minutes, and then replace it for another 20 minutes.

Apply hot compress

Warmth is extremely soothing, relaxes tight muscles, and increases blood flow. You can achieve it by applying a washcloth soaked in warm water, using a heating pad, or taking a hot shower or bath. If you are pregnant, however, consult your doctor before trying a hot soak.

Invest in a new mattress

A soft, sagging mattress may add up to the development of back problems or worsen an existing problem. However, if a new mattress is not a priority in your budget, a three-quarter-inch-thick piece of plywood placed between the mattress and box spring or frame may help somewhat.

Get some sleep

Getting sufficient rest at night plays a major role to ease strained back discomfort. It's best to lie on your side, with the knees flexed and a pillow between them. If you lie on your back, place a pillow under your knees.

Get a massage

If you're lucky enough to have an accommodating spouse, friend, roommate, or your masseuse, asks him or her to give you a rubdown. As you lie face down on a bed or sofa, ask him or her to knead your back muscles. Local massage therapists may also do home service if you can't visit one of them.

Relax

Much back pain is the product of muscles made tight caused by emotional tension. Master and practice the art of relaxation by doing meditation or trying a deep-breathing exercise, including closing your eyes, breathing slowly and deeply, and counting backward from 100.

Swim

Many experts believe that swimming is the best aerobic exercise for a bad back. Doing laps in the pool can shape up and strengthen your back and abdomen muscles, helping support the spine. While buoyancy temporarily eases your muscles of the job of holding up your weight, walking is the next best choice.

Watch your weight

Maintaining a healthy body weight (ask your doctor if you're not sure what that is) helps take the strain off the back muscles by lightening their load. What's more, having a flabby midsection may lead to having sway-backed, an abnormally hollow or sagging back, which can worsen an existing back pain.

Home Remedies from the Cupboard

Epsom salts

Epsom salts relieve back pain by reducing the inflammation. Fill your bathtub and add 2 cups salts. Soak for 30 minutes and relax.

Chamomile tea

Chamomile tea promotes a calming relief to soothe tense muscle tissue due to daily dress. During a break or after work, pamper yourself with a steaming mug. Steep a chamomile tea in 1 cup boiling water for 15 minutes. Drink 1-3 cups daily. Packaged tea may be safer to drink than tea made straightly from the flowers; as chamomile contains allergy-inducing proteins related to ragweed pollen. Confirm to your doctor if you are allergic to ragweed.

Rice

Fill a clean and thick sock with 1-cup uncooked rice, and then microwave it for about 30-60 seconds on medium-low heat. Check the temperature, if the heat is manageable, apply to your back.

Home Remedies from the Refrigerator

Milk

Bone up on milk. Women, especially, should include plenty of calcium in their diets. As women get older, the risk of having osteoporosis, the disease of eroding bones, becomes greater. Calcium promotes strong bones and gives protection to the spine from having osteoporosis.

Ginger Root

Ginger is not only effective on treating nausea but also back pain, as it contains anti-inflammatory compounds, including some with mild aspirin-like effects. When your back hurts, slice a 1- to 2-inch ginger root and add in 1-quart of boiling water. Simmer with lid on for 30 minutes over low heat. Cool for 30 minutes. Strain, sweeten with honey to taste, drink, and enjoy.

About The Author

Patrice St. Claire is a wife and a mom. She promotes active and healthy lifestyle, hence this book. Aside from writing books, she also enjoys "writing" codes for web developing. When she is not in front of the computer, she daydreams, eats, travels, photographs, and lives life to the fullest.

9 781986 257350